Autoimmune Protocol Cookbook:

Special Recipes for Breakfast, Lunch, dinner and Snacks

Dr. Susan M. Thomas

Table Of Content

Chapter One
Introduction to the Autoimmune Protocol

- What is the Autoimmune Protocol (AIP)?
- How does AIP differ from other diets?
- Benefits of the AIP diet
- AIP food list and guidelines

Chapter Two
Meal Planning and Preparation

- The importance of meal planning
- How to create an AIP grocery list
- Tips for food shopping on a budget
- Essential kitchen tools for AIP cooking

Chapter Three
Breakfast Recipes

- AIP-friendly breakfast ideas
- Recipes for egg-based dishes
- Recipes for grain-free porridges

- Recipes for smoothies and juices

Chapter Four
Snacks and Appetizers

- AIP-compliant snack ideas
- Recipes for dips and spreads
- Recipes for crackers and chips
- Recipes for bite-sized appetizers

Chapter Five
Main Dishes

- Recipes for meat-based dishes
- Recipes for seafood dishes
- Recipes for vegetarian and vegan options
- Recipes for stews, soups and casseroles

Chapter Six
Sides and Sauces

- Recipes for AIP-friendly vegetables dishes

Chapter One

Introduction to the Autoimmune Protocol

What is the Autoimmune Protocol (AIP)?

The Autoimmune Protocol (AIP) is a dietary regimen that lowers inflammation and encourages healing in patients with autoimmune illnesses. The AIP diet is a stringent, elimination-style diet that excludes particular foods and substances that contribute to autoimmune symptoms while simultaneously eating nutrient-dense, complete nutrition. The purpose of the AIP diet is to identify and remove the specific triggers that may produce signs and then carefully reintroduce foods to test whether they have a detrimental effect.

The AIP diet is based on the premise that specific foods might activate an immunological response in patients with autoimmune illnesses, leading to inflammation and worsening symptoms. These trigger fares might vary from person to person but usually include grains, legumes, dairy, soy, refined sugars, and processed meals. The AIP diet excludes certain trigger foods for some time, enabling the body to recover and minimize inflammation.

In addition to removing trigger foods, the AIP diet also promotes the intake of nutrient-dense, whole foods like vegetables, fruits, healthy fats, and high-quality meats and seafood. The idea is to supply the body with the nutrition it needs to recover while eliminating foods that may be causing damage.

It's crucial to emphasize that the AIP diet is not a permanent way of eating, and the objective is not to remain in the rigorous exclusion phase permanently. Instead, the aim is to identify and remove the precise triggers producing symptoms and then gently reintroduce meals to evaluate whether they have a detrimental effect. If a single item is discovered to trigger symptoms, it may be avoided in the long term, but many individuals can ultimately reintroduce a broad range of foods into their diet.

Overall, the Autoimmune Protocol is a dietary strategy that may be useful for persons with autoimmune illnesses since it tries to decrease inflammation and promote healing by removing trigger foods and integrating nutrient-dense, complete nutrition.

How does AIP differ from other diets?

The Autoimmune Protocol (AIP) is a unique dietary strategy that varies from many other diets in three significant ways:

Focus on inflammation reduction: Unlike many other diets, the principal purpose of the AIP diet is to decrease inflammation in the body and encourage healing for patients with autoimmune illnesses. This is done by removing trigger foods and introducing nutrient-dense, complete meals.

Rigorous elimination phase: The AIP diet begins with a strict elimination phase when particular foods and components that contribute to autoimmune symptoms are eliminated. This period might continue anywhere from a few weeks to months and is followed by a gradual reintroduction phase.

Whole food emphasis: The AIP diet promotes the eating of natural, nutrient-dense foods like vegetables, fruits, healthy fats, and high-quality meats and seafood. The idea is to supply the body with the nutrients it needs to repair while avoiding processed and refined meals.

Personalization: The AIP diet is exceptionally individualized since different people may have other trigger foods. The elimination phase and gradual reintroduction procedure help people to determine their unique trigger foods and adapt their diet appropriately.

Temporary elimination: Unlike other elimination diets, the purpose of the AIP diet is not to remain in the stringent elimination phase indefinitely. Instead, the goal is to identify and remove trigger meals and then gradually reintroduce a range of foods to evaluate whether they have a detrimental effect.

Compared to other diets, such as low-carb, low-fat, or vegan, the Autoimmune Protocol is highly personalized and focuses primarily on lowering inflammation and boosting healing for persons with autoimmune illnesses. While it might be more restricted compared to other diets, it can also be highly successful for persons with autoimmune disorders wanting to alleviate their symptoms through dietary modifications.

Benefits of the AIP diet

The Autoimmune Protocol (AIP) diet has been demonstrated to offer various advantages for patients with autoimmune illnesses, including:

Reduced inflammation: By removing trigger foods and introducing nutrient-dense, complete nutrition, the AIP diet may help reduce inflammation in the body, which is typically a key contributor to autoimmune symptoms.

Improved autoimmune symptoms: Many persons with autoimmune illnesses have experienced improvements in their symptoms, such as joint pain, tiredness, and skin concerns, after following the AIP diet.

Improved gut health: The AIP diet promotes the intake of nutrient-dense, whole foods, which may encourage the development of good gut flora and enhance gut health. A healthy gut is vital for general health and may also assist in easing autoimmune symptoms.

Increased nutritional intake: The AIP diet stresses the eating of nutrient-dense, whole foods, which may help guarantee the appropriate information of crucial vitamins and minerals, such as vitamins A, C, and D, and minerals like iron and magnesium.

Better food tolerance: By identifying and removing trigger foods, the AIP diet may assist persons with autoimmune illnesses in discovering which foods they tolerate well and which may be triggering symptoms. This may enhance general health and quality of life.

Enhanced energy: Many persons with autoimmune disorders have experienced increased energy levels after following the AIP diet, presumably due to better nutritional intake, lower inflammation, and improved gut health.

It's crucial to note that the advantages of the AIP diet may vary from person to person. People should consult a healthcare physician to establish whether the diet suits them and monitor their symptoms and progress. Additionally, the AIP diet is not a treatment for autoimmune illnesses but may be a helpful aid in controlling symptoms and improving general health.

AIP meal list and recommendations

The Autoimmune Protocol (AIP) diet is a whole-food-based, nutrient-dense diet that avoids specific foods and components considered to contribute to autoimmune symptoms. The following is a list of items commonly permitted and not allowed on the AIP diet:

1. Foods Allowed on the AIP Diet:

Vegetables: Leafy greens, root veggies, squash, and other non-starchy vegetables.
Fruits: Berries, melons, and other low-sugar fruits.

Meats: Grass-fed and pastured meats, poultry, and wild-caught fish.

Healthy fats: Coconut oil, olive oil, ghee, and other healthy fats.

Nuts and seeds: Soaked and sprouted nuts and seeds, such as almonds, walnuts, and sunflower seeds.

Herbs and spices: Fresh and dried herbs and spices, such as garlic, ginger, and turmeric.

2. Foods Not Allowed on the AIP Diet:

Grains: Wheat, barley, oats, maize, and other grains.

Legumes: Beans, lentils, and other legumes.

Dairy: Milk, cheese, and other dairy products.

Nightshade vegetables: Tomatoes, peppers, eggplants, and potatoes.

Processed and refined foods contain artificial preservatives, sweeteners, and other ingredients.

Eggs: Chicken eggs and various egg products.

Sugars: Refined and artificial sugars.

Alcohol: Wine, beer, and other alcoholic drinks.

The AIP diet is very customized, and some people may be able to tolerate some limited items after the first elimination phase. The progressive reintroduction phase is a critical element of the AIP diet, as it enables people to evaluate which foods they tolerate well and which may be producing problems.

In addition to the dietary restrictions, the AIP diet also contains advice for suitable lifestyle activities, such as obtaining proper sleep, avoiding stress, and participating in physical exercise.

It's crucial to understand that the AIP diet may be restrictive and require considerable food modifications. Individuals should engage with a healthcare physician to evaluate whether the diet suits them and monitor their symptoms and progress.

Chapter Two

Meal Planning and Preparation

The significance of meal planning

Meal planning is essential to following the Autoimmune Protocol (AIP) diet. It can help ensure that individuals get adequate nutrition, stick to the diet, and reduce stress and decision-making regarding mealtime. Some of the benefits of meal planning include the following:

Improved nutrient intake: Meal planning can help individuals ensure that they are consuming a balanced and nutrient-dense diet, which is essential for overall health and can help improve autoimmune symptoms.

Increased convenience: Having a plan for meals and snacks can make it easier to stick to the AIP diet, particularly on the move or when feasts are rapidly approaching.

Reduced stress: Meal preparation may minimize the stress and decision-making that typically accompany mealtime, enabling people to concentrate on other essential elements of their day.

Improved budgeting: Meal planning may help consumers save money by eliminating the need for impulsive purchases and allowing for bulk buying of goods.

Increased food diversity: Meal planning may help people include a variety of foods and tastes into their diet, guarantee proper nutritional intake, and make meals more pleasurable.

When it concerns meal preparation for the AIP diet, people may start by choosing their favorite AIP-friendly foods and meals and constructing a meal plan based on those items. Preparing snacks and having easy and fast supper alternatives for hectic days is also good.

It's crucial to remember that meal planning is a personal process, and what works well for one individual may not work for another. Individuals should feel free to experiment and alter their eating plans as required. Additionally, the AIP diet may involve additional time and work for meal preparation, particularly in the beginning. Still, the long-term advantages for general health and well-being may be well worth it.

Improved nutrient intake

Improved nutrient intake is one of the primary advantages of meal planning, especially when following the Autoimmune Protocol (AIP) diet. A well-planned AIP diet may supply a wide variety of critical nutrients, including vitamins, minerals, and healthy fats, that promote general health and help improve autoimmune symptoms.

Some of the critical nutrients that may be enhanced by meal planning on the AIP diet include:

Fiber: Fiber is crucial for digestive health and may help manage blood sugar levels. Foods such as leafy greens, root vegetables, and soaked and sprouted nuts and seeds are rich sources of fiber in the AIP diet.

Vitamins and minerals: Vitamins and minerals, such as vitamins A, C, D, and E, and minerals like magnesium and iron, are required for activities and may be provided via a balanced and nutrient-dense AIP diet.

Healthy fats: Healthy fats, such as those found in coconut oil, olive oil, and ghee, are vital for general health and may also help reduce inflammation, which is a typical concern for those with autoimmune diseases.

Protein: Protein is needed for developing and repairing tissues and may be gained from eating grass-fed and pastured meats, poultry, and wild-caught seafood.

By including a range of nutrient-dense foods into their diet and organizing meals properly, persons on the AIP diet may optimize their nutrient intake and promote their overall health. Additionally, meal planning helps people ensure that they receive enough of each vitamin and helps discover any nutritional deficiencies that need to be addressed.

Increased convenience

Increased convenience is another significant advantage of meal planning, particularly when following the Autoimmune Protocol (AIP) diet. Meal preparation may make it simpler to keep to the diet, even while on the move or when supper is rapidly coming.

Some of the ways that meal planning might boost convenience include:

Reduced impulsive purchases: When people have a plan for their meals and snacks, they are less likely to make impulse purchases, which may save time and money.

Quick and easy meal alternatives: By having a meal plan, people may guarantee fast and straightforward meal options for busy days, eliminating the need for takeout or processed meals.

Reduced decision-making: Meal planning may minimize the stress and decision-making that typically precede mealtime, making it more straightforward for people to stay on the AIP diet and avoid enticing non-compliant items.

Time-saving: Meal planning may save time in the long term by minimizing the need to make several journeys to the grocery store or by lowering the time spent cooking meals and snacks.

Better organization: Meal planning may help folks keep organized and ensure they have all the items they need, making it simpler to adhere to the AIP diet.

Overall, meal planning may boost convenience and make it simpler for people to follow the AIP diet, especially when confronted with hectic schedules or unplanned occurrences. This may eventually lead to enhanced adherence to the diet and better health results.

Reduced stress

Reduced stress is a crucial advantage of meal planning, especially when following the Autoimmune Protocol (AIP) diet. Planning meals in advance may help people manage their time more efficiently, decrease decision-making, and guarantee that they have fast and straightforward meal alternatives accessible, even on hectic days.

Here are some ways that meal planning might help alleviate stress:

Reduced choice fatigue: Meal planning may help decrease mental tiredness from making too many daily decisions. By having a plan in place, people may spend less time thinking about what to eat and more time enjoying their meals.

Improved time management: Meal planning may help people manage their time more successfully, freeing up time for other activities and lowering the stress of feeling like there is not enough time in the day to get everything done.

Greater food prep: By having a plan in place, people may minimize the time and effort necessary to prepare meals and snacks, resulting in reduced stress and improved overall well-being.

Improved stress management: Meal planning may help people better manage stress by minimizing the burden of decision-making and ensuring that they have nutritious and delicious meal alternatives accessible, especially on hectic days.

Improved dietary adherence: By having a meal plan in place, people may better stick to the AIP diet and minimize the stress of wondering about what to eat or whether they are eating enough of the proper foods.

Overall, meal planning may help decrease stress by increasing time management, minimizing decision-making, and ensuring that people have fast and simple meal alternatives accessible, even on hectic days. By lowering pressure, people may feel calmer and more focused, which can improve their general health and well-being.

Improved budgeting

Improved budgeting is another significant advantage of meal planning, particularly when following the Autoimmune Protocol (AIP) diet. By preparing meals in advance, consumers may decrease impulsive purchases, waste, and expenditure on food.

Here are some ways that meal planning might aid with budgeting:

Reduced impulsive purchases: Meal planning may help minimize impulse purchases by ensuring consumers have a plan for their meals and snacks, minimizing the need to make unexpected purchases.

Reduced food waste: By having a meal plan, consumers may guarantee they buy just the foods they need, minimizing food waste and saving money.

Better use of leftovers: Meal planning may help people better use pieces, decreasing waste and saving money on food.

Reduced expenditure on convenience foods: Meal planning may help consumers minimize their spending on convenience foods, such as takeout or processed meals, by ensuring that they have fast and straightforward meal alternatives accessible, even on busy days.

Improved supermarket buying: Meal planning may help consumers make more educated and budget-conscious selections while grocery shopping, lowering the probability of overpaying for food.

Overall, meal planning can improve budgeting by avoiding impulsive purchases, waste, and overpaying for food. By improving budgeting, people may better manage their resources, leading to greater overall well-being and lower financial stress.

Increased food variety

Increased food diversity is another crucial advantage of meal planning, particularly when adopting the Autoimmune Protocol (AIP) diet. While the AIP diet may appear limiting, people may enjoy a broad range of tasty, nutritious, and nutrient-dense meals with proper meal planning.

Here are some ways that meal planning might assist in enhancing dietary variety:

Expanded recipe repertoire: Meal planning may help people broaden their repertoire by encouraging them to explore new dishes and ingredients. This may lead to more food diversity and a more satisfying eating experience.

Improved dietary adherence: By having a meal plan in place, people may better stick to the AIP diet, minimizing the probability of succumbing to non-compliant food choices and increasing the diversity of foods ingested.

Better use of seasonal foods: Meal planning may help consumers make the most of seasonal ingredients, leading to more food diversity and a more sustainable and budget-conscious eating philosophy.

More purposeful food choices: Meal planning might help people make more conscious choices, lowering the possibility of depending on convenience meals and increasing the diversity of foods ingested.

Reduced boredom: Meal planning may help reduce boredom by encouraging people to explore different recipes, ingredients, and cooking methods, resulting in improved food diversity and a more pleasurable eating experience.

Overall, meal planning may enhance food diversity by extending dish repertoire, boosting dietary adherence, making greater use of seasonal items, and minimizing boredom.

Increased meal diversity may contribute to higher nutritional intake, improved satiety, and a more pleasurable eating experience.

How to construct an AIP grocery list

A shopping list is vital to meal planning, particularly following the Autoimmune Protocol (AIP) diet. A well-planned shopping list may ensure that consumers have all the goods they need to cook nutritious, tasty, and compliant meals.

Here are some suggestions for building an AIP grocery list:

Plan your meals: Before generating your shopping list, plan your weekly meals. Consider your schedule, special occasions, and any dietary restrictions or preferences.

Make a list of ingredients: Write down everything you need for each dish, including spices, herbs, and seasonings.

Check your pantry: Before preparing your shopping list, check your pantry and refrigerator to see what foods you already have. This may help prevent food waste and save money.

Follow the AIP food list: When building your shopping list, stick to the AIP food list and recommendations. Avoid processed meals, grains, legumes, and dairy, and concentrate on nutrient-dense foods, such as vegetables, meats, and healthy fats.

Make a list of staples: Make a list of essential things that you regularly use, such as coconut oil, bone broth, and ghee, so that you can stock up when they're on sale.

Consider your local retailers: Consider the businesses where you do your shopping, including farmers' markets and specialized stores, and note any promotions or special discounts.

Take advantage of bulk purchasing: Consider bulk buying things, such as nuts, seeds, and dried fruits, to save money and decrease packaging waste.

By following these recommendations, you may construct an AIP shopping list to ensure you have all the products you need to produce nutritious, tasty, and compliant meals. Meal planning and a well-planned shopping list improve budgeting, enhance food variety, and decrease stress, leading to better overall health and well-being.

Tips for food buying on a budget

Food shopping on a budget may be challenging, particularly when following a specified diet like the Autoimmune Protocol (AIP) (AIP). However, with careful preparation and a few methods, enjoying nutritious and tasty meals is feasible while remaining within a budget.

Here are some recommendations for food purchasing on a budget when following the AIP diet:

Make a food plan: Establish a meal plan for the week. This will help you avoid impulsive purchases and ensure you have everything you need to cook healthy and tasty meals.

Create a shopping list: Make a grocery list of all the items you need, depending on your meal plan. This will help you remain inside your budget and prevent overpaying.

Shop in season: Buy seasonal produce, which is frequently less costly and tastier. This will also help you make the most of locally available foods and lessen your carbon impact.

Buy in bulk: When shopping for essentials like nuts, seeds, and dried fruits, buy in quantity to save money. Make careful you store bulk things appropriately to avoid spoiling.

Consider generic or store-brand items: Consider purchasing generic or store-brand products, which are typically cheaper than brand-name products and just as excellent.

Shop at cheap shops: Look for discount stores or discount sections at your local grocery store, where you may get savings on fresh produce and pantry goods.

Please take advantage of bargains: Keep an eye out for discounts and special offers, and stock up on things while they're on sale.

Produce your own: Consider developing a little kitchen garden where you may grow your herbs, veggies, and fruits.

By following these guidelines, you may save money on your grocery shopping while following the AIP diet. Remember to be flexible and confident to try new meals and dishes. With a bit of forethought and imagination, you can eat nutritious and tasty meals while keeping within your budget.

Essential kitchen utensils for AIP cooking

The correct kitchen utensils may make cooking and preparing meals more straightforward, efficient, and pleasurable. When following the Autoimmune Protocol (AIP) diet, some kitchen gadgets might be extremely useful in producing healthful, nutrient-dense meals.

Here are some necessary kitchen utensils for AIP cooking:

High-quality cutting board: A durable, high-quality cutting board is a crucial tool for preparing ingredients and making meal preparation simpler.

Decent knives: Invest in a good collection of knives, including a chef's knife, paring knife, and serrated knife. This will make cutting, slicing, and dicing more straightforward and exact.

Blender or food processor: A blender or food processor may be used to prepare purees, smoothies, and sauces, as well as to grind nuts and seeds into flour.

Immersion blender: An immersion blender may mix soups, sauces, and stews directly in the pot, saving time and decreasing cleaning.

Slow cooker: A slow cooker may be used to create soups, stews, and casseroles and is a practical method to make meals while you're at work or doing errands.

Dutch oven: A Dutch oven is a flexible pot used for sautéing, roasting, and slow-cooking, making it a must-have for AIP cooking.

Casserole dishes: Casserole dishes are a terrific method to create one-pot meals, such as casseroles and baked dishes, and may be used for cooking and serving.

Baking sheets: Baking sheets are vital for roasting veggies and baking proteins and may also be used for producing AIP-compliant snacks and desserts.

Stainless steel pots and pans: Invest in high-quality stainless steel pots and pans, which are durable, simple to clean, and don't contain any dangerous chemicals.

Owning this critical kitchen equipment makes AIP cooking more straightforward, more efficient, and more pleasurable. With the correct tools, you can produce healthful, tasty, and nutrient-dense meals that promote your health and well-being.

Chapter Three

Breakfast Recipes

AIP-friendly breakfast ideas

When following the Autoimmune Protocol (AIP) diet, breakfast may be a problem since many classic breakfast items are not permitted. However, you can make tasty, healthy, and AIP-friendly breakfast alternatives with ingenuity.

Here are some AIP-friendly breakfast ideas:

Sweet Potato and Apple Hash: Grate sweet potatoes, apples, and sauté with coconut oil, cinnamon, and ginger. Serve with a side of crispy bacon or sausage.

Avocado and Egg Breakfast Bowl: Mash one avocado and add chopped tomatoes, salt, and pepper. Top with a fried or poached egg and sprinkle with cilantro.

Veggie-Packed Omelet: Fill an omelet with sautéed veggies such as spinach, mushrooms, and onions. Top with avocado and salsa.

AIP Granola: Mix unsweetened coconut flakes, chopped nuts, seeds, and spices. Bake till crispy and serve with coconut milk or almond milk.

Berry and Banana Smoothie: Blend frozen berries, a banana, coconut milk, and a scoop of AIP-friendly protein powder.

AIP Pancakes: Mix almond flour, coconut flour, eggs, coconut milk, and a bit of salt. Cook in a non-stick pan and serve with sliced fruit and coconut oil.

Sweet Potato & Sausage Breakfast Bake: Layer sliced sweet potatoes, sausage, and any desired veggies in a baking dish. Bake until crispy and serve with eggs or avocado.

Chia Seed Pudding: Mix chia seeds, coconut milk, vanilla essence, and preferred sweeteners. Let it settle in the fridge overnight and serve with fruit in the morning.

With these AIP-friendly breakfast recipes, you can start your day with a healthy and tasty meal that promotes your health and well-being.

Additionally, you may be creative and tweak these recipes to fit your tastes and preferences. Remember to concentrate on nutrient-dense items and avoid processed meals, carbohydrates, and refined sugars.

Recipes for egg-based cuisine

Eggs are a mainstay in many AIP diets since they are flexible and nutrient-dense. Here are some egg-based foods that are compatible with the Autoimmune Protocol (AIP) diet:

AIP Frittata: Sauté a variety of veggies such as spinach, mushrooms, and onions. Mix in beaten eggs, salt, and pepper and bake until set.

Shakshuka:
1. Sauté tomatoes, onions, and spices in a skillet.
2. Make wells in the mixture and break eggs into them.
3. Cover the pan and simmer until the eggs are set.
4. Serve with sliced avocado.

AIP Quiche: Mix coconut flour, milk, eggs, salt, and any desired seasonings. Pour into a greased pie plate and pour in sautéed veggies and cooked meat. Bake until set.

AIP Eggs Benedict: Poach eggs and serve on top of AIP-friendly English muffins or roasted sweet potato slices. Top with AIP-friendly hollandaise sauce and sliced ham or bacon.

AIP Breakfast Burrito: Fill a big lettuce leaf with scrambled eggs, chopped veggies, and avocado. Roll up and serve with salsa.

AIP Scrambled Eggs: Scramble eggs with coconut oil and any preferred seasonings. Serve with sliced avocado and sautéed veggies.

AIP Omelet: Fill with sautéed veggies, cooked meat, and preferred herbs and spices. Serve with sliced avocado and a side of fruit.

These egg-based recipes are tasty and offer a decent dose of protein, healthy fats, and vitamins and minerals to support your overall health and well-being. You may also be creative and adapt these recipes to suit your taste preferences. Remember to concentrate on nutrient-dense items and avoid processed meals, carbohydrates, and refined sugars.

AIP Frittata

An AIP Frittata is a baked egg dish consistent with the Autoimmune Protocol (AIP) diet. Here's how you can create a simple AIP Frittata:

Ingredients:

- 6-8 eggs
- 1-2 teaspoons of coconut oil
- 2 cups of diced veggies (such as spinach, mushrooms, onions, bell peppers, etc.) (such as spinach, mushrooms, onions, bell peppers, etc.)
- Salt and pepper to taste

Instructions:

1. Warm the oven to 375°F (190°C).

2. In a large oven-safe pan, heat the coconut oil over medium heat.

3. Add the diced veggies and simmer until softened, approximately 5-7 minutes.

4. In a separate dish, beat the eggs with salt and pepper.

5. Pour the beaten eggs over the veggies in the pan. Stir carefully to spread the eggs evenly.

6. Put the pan in the oven and toast for 10-12 minutes or until the eggs are set.

7. Retrieve the pan from the oven and allow it to cool for a few minutes.

8. Slice the frittata and serve hot.

The AIP Frittata is a terrific way to start your day or have a tasty and healthy lunch or supper. You may be creative and add other veggies, meats, or spices to suit your taste preferences. You can also serve the frittata with a side of fruit or a salad for a well-rounded dinner. Remember to concentrate on nutrient-dense items and avoid processed meals, carbohydrates, and refined sugars.

Shakshuka

Shakshuka is a typical Middle Eastern meal that consists of eggs poached in a delicious tomato sauce. It is a simple and tasty recipe consistent with the Autoimmune Protocol (AIP) diet. Here's how you can create a simple AIP Shakshuka:

Ingredients:

- Two teaspoons of coconut oil
- One onion, chopped
- Three garlic cloves minced
- Two bell peppers, diced \s2 tomatoes, diced
- One teaspoon of ground cumin
- One teaspoon of paprika
- Salt and pepper to taste
- 4-6 eggs
- Fresh parsley or cilantro, chopped (optional) (optional)
- Sliced avocado (optional) (optional)

Instructions:

1. In a large pan, heat the coconut oil over medium heat.

2. Add the chopped onion and minced garlic and heat until softened, approximately 5 minutes.

3. Add the chopped bell peppers and continue cooking for another 5 minutes.

4. Stir in the diced tomatoes, ground cumin, paprika, salt, and pepper. Let the ingredients boil for 10-15 minutes or until the sauce has thickened.

5. Make wells in the sauce with a spoon and break the eggs into them.

6. Cover the pan and let the eggs simmer for approximately 5-7 minutes or until the whites are set, but the yolks are still runny.

7. Serve the shakshuka hot with chopped parsley or cilantro and sliced avocado (if preferred) (if desired).

The AIP Shakshuka is a tasty and gratifying dinner that can be eaten any day. You may also tweak the recipe to suit your taste preferences by adding various spices or veggies. Remember to concentrate on nutrient-dense items and avoid processed meals, carbohydrates, and refined sugars.

AIP Quiche

An AIP Quiche is a baked egg dish consistent with the Autoimmune Protocol (AIP) diet. Here's how you can create a simple AIP Quiche:

Ingredients:

- 6-8 eggs
- 1 cup of full-fat coconut milk
- One teaspoon of salt

- One teaspoon of black pepper
- 2 cups of diced veggies (such as spinach, mushrooms, onions, bell peppers, etc.) (such as spinach, mushrooms, onions, bell peppers, etc.)
- One tablespoon of coconut oil
- Herbs (which including parsley, thyme, or basil) (such as parsley, thyme, or basil)

Instructions:

1. Warm the oven to 375°F (190°C).

2. In a large oven-safe pan, heat the coconut oil over medium heat.

3. Add the diced veggies and simmer until softened, approximately 5-7 minutes.

4. In a separate dish, beat the eggs with coconut milk, salt, and pepper.

5. Stir in the cooked veggies and any desired herbs.

6. Pour the mixture into a 9-inch (23 cm) pie plate.

7. Put the dish in the oven and bake for 25-30 minutes or until the eggs are set, and the top is golden brown.

8. Remove the dish from the oven and let it cool for a few minutes.

9. Serve the quiche hot or cold.

The AIP Quiche is a terrific way to have a tasty and nutritious dinner full of veggies, healthy fats, and protein. You may be creative and add other veggies, meats, or spices to suit your taste preferences. You can also serve the quiche with a side of fruit or a salad for a well-rounded dinner. Remember to concentrate on nutrient-dense items and avoid processed meals, carbohydrates, and refined sugars.

Eggs Benedict is a popular brunch meal that may be altered to be consistent with the Autoimmune Protocol (AIP) diet. Here's how you can prepare AIP Eggs Benedict:

Ingredients:

- 2-4 eggs
- Four pieces of AIP-friendly bread (such as coconut flour bread or plantain bread) (such as coconut flour bread or plantain bread)
- Four slices of ham or other AIP-friendly meat
- One avocado
- Two teaspoons of lemon juice
- Salt & pepper, to taste
- Fresh herbs (such as parsley, thyme, or basil) (such as parsley, thyme, or basil)

Instructions:

1. Fill a big pot with water and bring to a medium simmer.

2. Crack each egg into a minor basin and gently pour each egg into the heating water.

3. Cook the eggs for 3-5 minutes or until the whites are set, but the yolks are still runny.

4. Remove the eggs from the water with a slotted spoon and put them aside on a dish lined with paper towels.

5. Toast the bread till golden brown.

6. Mash the avocado with lemon juice and season with salt and pepper.

7. Spread the avocado mixture on top of each piece of bread.

8. Top each piece of bread with a slice of ham.

9. Put a scrambled egg on top of each piece of ham.

10. Sprinkle with fresh herbs and serve immediately.

The AIP Eggs Benedict is a tasty and fulfilling meal with a nice mix of protein, healthy fats, and carbs. The avocado gives healthy fats, the eggs supply protein, and the bread and ham provide carbs. This meal may be a terrific way to start your day or to enjoy it as a brunch treat. You may be creative with the toppings and use other meats, veggies, or herbs to suit your taste preferences. Remember to concentrate on nutrient-dense items and avoid processed meals, carbohydrates, and refined sugars.

AIP Breakfast Burrito

A Breakfast Burrito is a delightful and handy way to start your day and can be readily changed to be consistent with the Autoimmune Protocol (AIP) diet. Here's how you can prepare an AIP Breakfast Burrito:

Ingredients:

- 2-4 eggs
- 2-4 teaspoons of coconut oil or other AIP-friendly oil
- One onion, diced
- One red bell pepper, chopped
- 1-2 cloves of garlic, minced
- Salt & pepper, to taste
- 1-2 teaspoons of fresh herbs (such as parsley, thyme, or cilantro), chopped \s4-8 slices of AIP-friendly meat (such as ham, bacon, or sausage) (such as ham, bacon, or link)
- 4-8 AIP-friendly wraps (such as lettuce leaves, collard greens, or nori sheets)

(such as lettuce leaves, collard greens, or nori sheets)

Instructions:

1. In a medium saucepan, simmer the oil over medium high heat.

2. Add the onion and red pepper to the pan and simmer for 5-7 minutes, until tender.

3. Add the garlic to the pan and simmer for 1-2 minutes, until fragrant.

4. Crack the eggs into the skillet and scramble until completely done.

5. Season the eggs with salt, pepper, and fresh herbs.

6. Cook the AIP-friendly meat in a separate pan until crispy.

7. Place an AIP-friendly wrap on a dish and pour a liberal amount of the egg mixture into the Middle.

8. Top with a slice of cooked meat.

9. Roll up the wrap and enjoy!

The AIP Breakfast Burrito is a filling and nutritious meal that provides a good balance of protein, healthy fats, and carbohydrates. The eggs and meat provide protein, while the wrap and vegetables provide carbohydrates. This meal may be a terrific way to start your day or enjoy a quick, straightforward breakfast. You may be creative with the ingredients and add various veggies, herbs, or spices to suit your taste preferences. Remember to concentrate on nutrient-dense items and avoid processed meals, carbohydrates, and refined sugars.

Recipes for grain-free porridges

Grain-free porridges are a tasty and healthy way to start your day and are consistent with the Autoimmune Protocol (AIP) diet. Here are a few AIP-friendly recipes for grain-free porridges:

Sweet Potato Porridge:

Ingredients:

- Two medium-sized sweet potatoes, peeled and diced
- 2 cups of coconut milk
- One teaspoon of cinnamon
- 1/4 teaspoon of nutmeg
- 1/4 teaspoon of sea salt
- Optional toppings: chopped nuts, dried fruit, and coconut flakes

Instructions:

1. Add sweet potatoes, coconut milk, cinnamon, nutmeg, and sea salt in a large saucepan.

2. Bring the mixture to a simmer and then lower the heat to low.

3. Simmer the mixture for 20-30 minutes, stirring periodically, until the sweet potatoes are tender and the liquid is thick and creamy.

4. Pour the mixture into bowls and top with your favorite toppings.

5. Coconut Milk Porridge:

Ingredients:

- 2 cups of coconut milk
- 1 cup of coconut flakes
- 1/4 teaspoon of cinnamon

- 1/4 teaspoon of sea salt
- Optional toppings: chopped nuts, dried fruit, and coconut flakes

Instructions:

1. Add coconut milk, coconut flakes, cinnamon, and sea salt in a large saucepan.

2. Bring the mixture to a simmer and then lower the heat to low.

3. Simmer the mixture for 10-15 minutes, stirring regularly, until the liquid is thick and creamy.

4. Pour the mixture into bowls and top with your favorite toppings.

These grain-free porridges are a pleasant and nutrient-dense alternative to regular oatmeal and offer a nice mix of carbs, healthy fats, and protein. Sweet potatoes and coconut milk are excellent sources of vitamins, minerals, and antioxidants, while the toppings hint at sweetness and crunch. These simple porridges may be a terrific way to start your day or enjoy a quick and fulfilling breakfast. You may be creative with the ingredients and add other spices, herbs, or sweeteners to suit your taste preferences. Remember to concentrate on nutrient-dense items and avoid processed meals, carbohydrates, and refined sugars.

Recipes for smoothies and liquids

Smoothies and juices are a practical and tasty way to receive a rapid burst of nutrients and can be readily made AIP-compliant. Here are a few AIP-friendly recipes for smoothies and juices:

Green Smoothie:

Ingredients:

- 2 cups of spinach

- 1 cup of coconut milk
- One banana
- 1/2 avocado
- 1/4 teaspoon of cinnamon
- 1/4 teaspoon of sea salt
- Optional sweetener: 1 tablespoon of honey or maple syrup

Instructions:

1. Add the spinach, coconut milk, banana, avocado, cinnamon, sea salt, and any sweetener in a blender.

2. Blend the ingredients until smooth and creamy.

3. Pour the mixture into glasses and enjoy immediately.

4. Carrot-Ginger Juice:

Ingredients:

- Four medium-sized carrots, peeled and cut
- 1/2 inch of fresh ginger, peeled and chopped
- 1/2 lemon, juiced
- 1/4 teaspoon of sea salt

Instructions:

1. Add carrots, ginger, lemon juice, and sea salt in a juicer.

2. Juice the mixture until all the components are mixed.

3. Pour the mixture into glasses and enjoy immediately.

These smoothies and juices are a terrific way to add additional nutrients to your diet and are simple to mix and adapt to your taste preferences. They are a fantastic way to have a fast and enjoyable snack or to enjoy as part of a bigger meal. When creating smoothies and juices, concentrate on nutrient-dense ingredients and avoid processed foods, grains, and refined sugars. Also, remember that too many smoothies and juices might increase sugar intake, so it's better to enjoy them in moderation.

Chapter Four

Snacks and Appetizers

AIP-compliant snack ideas

Snacks are an excellent way to keep your energy levels up throughout the day, particularly if following the Autoimmune Protocol (AIP) diet. Here are a few AIP-compliant snack options that you may enjoy:

Vegetable sticks with guacamole or hummus: Cut up carrots, cucumbers, celery, or other veggies into bars and serve with homemade guacamole or hummus prepared with AIP-compliant foods.

AIP-friendly food: Fresh fruit such as berries, apples, or pears make a fantastic, healthful snack. Avoid dried fruits, which may be heavy in sugar and difficult to digest.

AIP-friendly nuts and seeds: Nuts such as almonds, walnuts, and macadamia nuts, and seeds such as sunflower seeds, pumpkin seeds, and chia seeds make a terrific, crunchy snack. Just be careful to avoid roasted or salted types, which might contain dangerous ingredients.

AIP-compliant trail mix: Mix AIP-friendly nuts, seeds, dried fruit, and coconut flakes for a fast and tasty snack.

AIP-friendly crackers: Make your crackers using AIP-compliant items like coconut flour, cassava flour, or almond flour. Serve with guacamole or hummus for dipping.

AIP-friendly smoothies or juices: Make a fast and straightforward smoothie or juice with AIP-compliant products for a nutrient-dense snack.

AIP-compliant jerky: Make your jerky from AIP-compliant sources such as turkey, beef, or salmon, or buy AIP-friendly jerky products at a health food shop.

When picking snacks, it's vital to concentrate on nutrient-dense foods and avoid processed or refined meals. Aim to consume various snacks to ensure you're receiving a balanced intake of nutrients.

Recipes for dips and spreads

Dips and spreads are a terrific way to add flavor and diversity to your meals, mainly if you follow the Autoimmune Protocol (AIP) diet. Here are a few AIP-compliant recipes for dips and spreads:

Guacamole: Made with ripe avocados, fresh lime juice, salt, and other AIP-compliant ingredients, guacamole is a tasty and healthful dip. Serve with veggie sticks or crackers.

Hummus: Made from chickpeas, tahini, garlic, and lemon juice, hummus is a popular spread that may be made AIP-friendly by utilizing AIP-compliant components. Serve with veggie sticks or crackers.

AIP-friendly pesto: Made with fresh basil, AIP-compliant nuts such as almonds or pine nuts, garlic, and olive oil, pesto is a tasty spread that may be used as a sauce or space.

Olive tapenade: Made with olives, capers, lemon juice, and olive oil, olive tapenade is a tangy and savory spread that's excellent for crackers or toast.

AIP-compliant salsa: Made with fresh tomatoes, onion, lime juice, and other AIP-compliant ingredients, salsa is a delightful dip that's ideal for chips or tacos.

AIP-friendly tzatziki: Made with coconut yogurt, cucumber, garlic, and lemon juice, tzatziki is a creamy and delicious dip that's excellent for pita bread or crackers.

These recipes may be readily altered to your preference, and you can experiment with various components to discover your ideal mix. Just stick to AIP-compliant items and avoid processed or refined meals.

Recipes for crackers and chips

Crackers and chips may be a fantastic snack or supplement to a meal on the Autoimmune Protocol (AIP) diet; however, regular crackers and chips frequently include grains and other items that are not AIP-compliant. Here are some AIP-friendly recipes for crackers and chips:

Plantain chips: Thinly sliced and baked or fried, plantains produce a tasty and crispy snack that may be seasoned with AIP-compliant seasonings.

Sweet potato chips: Thinly sliced and baked or fried sweet potatoes produce a tasty and healthful snack that's excellent for dipping in AIP-friendly dips.

Cassava chips: Made from cassava flour, these chips are crispy, gluten-free, and AIP-compliant. They may be seasoned with AIP-compliant seasonings for added taste.

Coconut chips: Made from unsweetened coconut flakes, they are crispy and crunchy, making a fantastic snack or addition to salads.

AIP crackers: Made from AIP-compliant flours such as almond or cassava flour, these crackers are gluten-free and may be seasoned with AIP-compliant seasonings.

Zucchini chips: Thinly sliced and baked, zucchini produces a crispy and nutritious chip that's excellent for snacking or as a side dish.

When preparing your crackers and chips, use high-quality, fresh ingredients and avoid processed or refined items. Additionally, always check the labels on any store-bought crackers or chips to be sure they are AIP-compliant.

Plantain chips

Plantain chips are a popular and tasty snack consistent with the Autoimmune Protocol (AIP) diet. Plantains are starchy fruit similar to bananas but are more complex and have lower sugar content.

To prepare plantain chips, start peeling and slicing 2-3 ripe plantains into thin rounds. Then, heat a few teaspoons of oil in a big skillet over medium heat, and add the plantain slices in a single layer. Fry until golden brown, rotating once, then remove from the pan using a slotted spoon to drain on a paper towel. Sprinkle with salt or other AIP-compliant spices, if preferred.

Plantain chips may be refrigerated in an airtight container for up to a week, and they make a terrific snack on their own or as a side dish with dips. They are also a healthier alternative to typical potato chips since they are lower in sugar and carbs and include fiber and minerals such as vitamin C and potassium.

Coconut chips

Coconut chips are a crispy and tasty snack consistent with the Autoimmune Protocol (AIP) diet. Coconut chips are formed from unsweetened coconut flakes that have been roasted or dried till crispy.

To produce coconut chips:
1. Warm your oven to 350°F (175°C).
2. Spread a single layer of unsweetened coconut flakes on a baking sheet, and bake for 10-15 minutes or until golden brown and crispy.

3. Be cautious about mixing the flakes every
   5 minutes to achieve consistent heating
   and to avoid burning.

Coconut chips are a fantastic snack on their own, or they may be added to salads, smoothies, and other foods for a crunchy texture and a bit of coconut flavor. They are also an excellent source of healthful fats, fiber, and minerals such as iron and magnesium.

When buying coconut chips, be sure to purchase unsweetened and unflavored versions since many store-bought coconut chips have added sugar and other additives that are not AIP-compliant. Additionally, carefully examine the ingredient list for any added additives, such as preservatives or stabilizers, that may not be AIP-friendly.

AIP crackers

AIP crackers are a crispy and tasty snack consistent with the Autoimmune Protocol (AIP) diet. Unlike ordinary crackers manufactured with wheat flour, AIP crackers are often prepared with nut flours, such as almond or coconut flour, and are seasoned with AIP-friendly herbs and spices.

To create AIP crackers, combine the ingredients in a bowl, roll out the dough on a sheet of parchment paper, and then cut it into pieces. Bake in a preheated oven until crispy and golden brown, which generally takes approximately 15-20 minutes.

Some typical components used in AIP crackers are almond flour, coconut flour, olive oil, eggs, salts, and AIP-compliant herbs and spices, such as rosemary or thyme. For added taste and texture, you may also toss in other ingredients, like chopped veggies or nuts.

AIP crackers are a fantastic snack on their own, or they may be coupled with dips, spreads, and other AIP-compliant snack items. They are also a tremendous source of healthy fats, fiber, and protein and a quick and portable snack alternative.

Zucchini chips

Zucchini chips are a nutritious and tasty snack consistent with the Autoimmune Protocol (AIP) diet. They are produced by thinly slicing zucchini and then baking or dehydrating them till crispy.

To create zucchini chips, clean and slice zucchini into thin rounds. Place the pieces in a single layer on a baking sheet or a dehydrator tray, and then season with salt, pepper, and any AIP-compliant herbs and spices. Bake in a warm oven at 375°F (190°C) for 20-25 minutes or until the chips are golden brown and crispy. Alternatively, you may dry the slices for 8-12 hours in a dehydrator until they are crisp and flaky.

Zucchini chips are a fantastic snack on their own, or they may be coupled with dips, spreads, and other AIP-compliant snack items. They are also an excellent source of vitamins and minerals, such as vitamins C and A, and potassium. Additionally, zucchini chips are low in calories and carbs, making them a fantastic snack choice for individuals following a low-carb or AIP diet.

Recipes for bite-sized appetizers

Bite-sized appetizers are compact, tasty meals that are excellent for entertaining or eating. Numerous wonderful and AIP-compliant recipes for bite-sized appetizers are simple to create and delightful to consume. Here are a few examples:

AIP Meatballs: Made using ground meat, such as beef or pig, and seasoned with herbs and spices like garlic, ginger, and turmeric. Serve them with a tasty dipping sauce for a pleasant snack.

AIP Stuffed Dates: Dates are filled with almond butter or coconut cream and then topped with bacon or chopped nuts for a sweet and salty snack.

AIP Vegetable Crudités: A variety of vegetables, such as carrots, cucumbers, and bell peppers, are sliced and served with a dipping sauce made from AIP-compliant ingredients like coconut cream or avocado.

AIP Deviled Eggs: Hard-boiled eggs are sliced in half, and the yolks are mashed with AIP-friendly ingredients like avocado or coconut cream, then piped back into the egg whites for a creamy and satisfying snack.

AIP Seafood Cakes: Fresh seafood, such as crab or shrimp, is mixed with herbs, spices, and coconut flour to make delicious and flavorful cakes that are perfect for snacking or as an appetizer.

These recipes and others like them are a great way to enjoy the flavors and benefits of AIP-compliant foods while still indulging in delicious and satisfying snacks and appetizers.

Chapter Five

Main Dishes

Recipes for meat-based dishes

Meat-based dishes are a staple of the AIP diet, providing essential nutrients and protein. There are many delicious and AIP-compliant recipes for meat-based dishes that are easy to prepare and perfect for any meal of the day. Here are a few examples:

AIP Slow Cooker Pork Roast: Pork roast is slow-cooked with herbs and spices like garlic, rosemary, and thyme for a delicious and tender main dish.

AIP Chicken Curry: Chicken is simmered in a flavorful sauce made from coconut milk, turmeric, ginger, and other AIP-friendly spices.

AIP Beef Stir-Fry - Thinly sliced beef is stir-fried with vegetables like bell peppers and onions and seasoned with herbs and spices like ginger and garlic.

AIP Lamb Chops: Lamb chops are seasoned with herbs and spices like rosemary and thyme, then grilled or baked for a delicious and easy main dish.

AIP Baked Salmon: Salmon is baked with lemon, herbs, and spices for a tasty and healthful main meal.

These and other meat-based recipes are a terrific way to experience the advantages of the AIP diet while still indulging in tasty and gratifying main courses. By incorporating herbs, spices, and other AIP-compliant ingredients, these meals will likely become favorites in your meal rotation.

AIP Slow Cooker Pork Roast

AIP Slow Cooker Pork Roast is a tasty and easy-to-make main meal appropriate for the autoimmune protocol (AIP) diet. This dish is produced by slow-cooking pork roast with herbs and spices, including garlic, rosemary, and thyme. The lengthy cooking procedure helps to tenderize the beef and infuse it with taste, while the herbs and spices offer further depth and richness.

To prepare AIP Slow Cooker Pork Roast, you will need the following ingredients:

- Pork roast
- Garlic, minced
- Rosemary, dried
- Thyme, dry
- Salt
- Black pepper
- Coconut oil or other AIP-compliant fat

Instructions:

1. Season the pork roast with salt, black pepper, and chopped garlic.

2. Add a layer of herbs like rosemary and thyme in a slow cooker.

3. Place the seasoned pork roast in the slow cooker on top of the herbs.

4. Drizzle the roast with melted coconut oil or other AIP-compliant fat.

5. Grill on low for 8-10 hours or until the roast is tender and cooked through.

6. Serve the pork roast with your favorite AIP-compliant sides like roasted veggies or a salad.

This meal is a terrific way to experience the advantages of the AIP diet while still having a tasty and fulfilling main dish. The lengthy cooking procedure guarantees that the meat is soft and delicious, while the herbs and spices provide depth and richness to the meal. With its essential ingredients and easy-to-follow directions, this dish is a terrific choice for anybody trying to integrate more AIP-friendly foods into their diet.

AIP Chicken Curry

AIP Chicken Curry is a tasty and healthy recipe appropriate for the autoimmune protocol (AIP) diet. This recipe uses a blend of fragrant spices, tender chicken, and a creamy coconut milk-based sauce to make a delightful and fulfilling main meal.

To create AIP Chicken Curry, you will need the following ingredients:

- Chicken breast, cubed
- Onion, diced
- Garlic, minced

- Ginger, grated
- Turmeric powder
- Cumin powder
- Coriander powder
- Sea salt
- Black pepper
- Coconut milk
- Coconut oil or other AIP-compliant fat

Instructions:

1. Heat a big saucepan over medium heat and add coconut oil or other AIP-compliant fat.

2. Add the chopped onion, minced garlic, and grated ginger to the pan and heat until the onion is tender and translucent.

3. Add the turmeric powder, cumin powder, coriander powder, salt, and pepper to the pan and stir to mix.

4. Add the cubed chicken to the pan and cook until browned on both sides.

5. Pour in the coconut milk and whisk to mix.

6. Reduce heat to low, cover the pan, and allow the curry to simmer for 15-20 minutes or until the chicken is thoroughly cooked and tender.

7. Serve the AIP Chicken Curry hot over a bed of steamed veggies or with a side of roasted sweet potatoes.

This meal is a terrific way to enjoy the tastes and benefits of the AIP diet while still having a tasty and fulfilling main dinner.

It's also a flexible recipe that can be readily altered to your tastes and preferences. For example, you may add other veggies, such as carrots, bell peppers, or kale, to boost the nutritious value of the meal. You may also vary the spice level by adding more or fewer spices used in the recipe.

AIP Beef Stir-Fry

AIP Beef Stir-Fry is a fast and simple dinner that's excellent for hectic weeknights. It's created using thin slices of beef, such as flank steak or sirloin, that are stir-fried with veggies like broccoli, carrots, and onion. The meat is seasoned with AIP-compliant spices, such as ginger, garlic, and coconut aminos, and then stir-fried until it's browned and cooked. This meal is hearty, tasty, and rich in nutrients, making it an excellent alternative for individuals following the autoimmune protocol diet.

One of the nice things about AIP Beef Stir-Fry is that you can personalize it to your desire. For example, you may add additional veggies, such as zucchini, mushrooms, or bell peppers, to improve the fiber and nutritious value of the meal. You may also vary the spiciness level by using more or less of the different spices used in the recipe. Additionally, you can serve the stir-fry over a bed of cauliflower rice or other AIP-compliant grain-free grains to make it a complete meal.

AIP Lamb Chops

AIP Lamb Chops is a tasty and healthy recipe for special occasions or when you want a robust and fulfilling supper. It's cooked with lamb chops seasoned with AIP-compliant herbs and spices, such as rosemary, thyme, and garlic, and then grilled or pan-fried to perfection.

One of the nice things about AIP Lamb Chops is that they're high in critical nutrients, like protein, iron, and healthy fats. Additionally, lamb is an excellent source of zinc, which is crucial for immune function and skin health. When coupled with AIP-compliant sides, such as roasted vegetables or a salad, AIP Lamb Chops make for a complete and balanced dinner.

When creating AIP Lamb Chops, buying a high-quality, grass-fed, and pastured lamb is crucial for the most incredible flavor and nutritional profile. Additionally, make sure to cook the lamb to your chosen degree of doneness, whether medium-rare, medium, or well-done. This meal may be eaten on its own or served with several AIP-friendly condiments, such as fresh herbs, lemon juice, or a simple sauce prepared with coconut milk.

AIP Baked Salmon

AIP Baked Salmon is a simple and tasty recipe that's excellent for a weekday supper or entertaining guests. Baking salmon fillets are produced in the oven with AIP-compliant spices, such as lemon juice, garlic, and fresh herbs. The result is a delicate and tasty fish rich in omega-3 fatty acids, protein, and other critical elements.

One of the nice things about AIP Baked Salmon is that it's simple to cook and can be adjusted to fit your taste preferences. For example, you may use flavors like dill or basil or add things like chopped vegetables or fruit to the baking dish.

Additionally, you may use other cooking techniques, such as grilling or pan-frying, to generate varied textures and tastes.

When creating AIP Baked Salmon, buying high-quality, wild-caught salmon is crucial for the most outstanding flavor and nutritional profile. Additionally, be careful to bake the salmon for the exact time since overcooking might result in dry and challenging fish. This meal may have several AIP-friendly sides, such as roasted vegetables, sweet potato mash, or a salad. Whether you're a lover of salmon or simply looking for a fast and healthy supper, AIP Baked Salmon is a tasty and nutritious alternative.

Recipes for seafood meals

The Autoimmune Protocol (AIP) diet provides several seafood selections that are tasty and nutritionally healthy. Seafood is a high source of omega-3 fatty acids, which are needed for healthy brain function and decreasing inflammation. Additionally, seafood is abundant in protein and other vital elements, making it a crucial component of the AIP diet.

Here are some AIP-friendly seafood meals that you may include in your meal planning:

AIP Shrimp Scampi: Shrimp is a quick-cooking seafood alternative that's excellent for hectic weeknights. AIP Shrimp Scampi is cooked by sautéing shrimp in coconut oil with garlic, lemon juice, and AIP-compliant herbs for a tasty and fulfilling meal.

AIP Crab Cakes: Crab cakes are a popular seafood meal that may be readily adapted to the AIP diet. To prepare AIP crab cakes, use almond flour instead of breadcrumbs, and season with lemon juice, Old Bay seasoning, and AIP-compliant herbs.

AIP Clam Chowder: Clam chowder is a substantial and soothing soup that's excellent for chilly times. To prepare an AIP-friendly version, use coconut cream instead of dairy and add AIP-compliant veggies, such as leeks and carrots, for extra taste and nutrients.

AIP Grilled Salmon: Grilled salmon is a simple and tasty recipe that's excellent for summer picnics. Season the salmon with AIP-compliant spices, such as paprika and cumin, and grill until just cooked. Serve with grilled veggies and a lemon slice for a full supper.

AIP Lobster Bisque: Lobster bisque is a delicious and indulgent soup that's excellent for special occasions. To prepare an AIP-friendly version, use coconut cream instead of dairy, and add AIP-compliant veggies, such as leeks and fennel, for extra taste and nutrients.

Whether you're a lover of shrimp, crab, or lobster, there are several AIP-friendly seafood recipes to select from. Incorporating seafood into your AIP diet enhances your nutritional intake, promotes dietary variety, and offers a tasty and fulfilling source of protein.

AIP Shrimp Scampi

AIP Shrimp Scampi is a delectable seafood meal acceptable for the Autoimmune Protocol (AIP) diet. This meal typically consists of giant shrimp sautéed in a blend of garlic, coconut oil, lemon juice, and fresh herbs. The sauce is rich and creamy, and the shrimp are cooked until they become pink.

This dish is generally served over a bed of spaghetti squash or zucchini noodles for a gluten-free and grain-free supper. Some variants of AIP Shrimp Scampi may include using coconut cream for extra richness or ghee instead of coconut oil for a more traditional taste. Overall, this meal is a tasty and nutritious alternative for individuals following the AIP diet since it includes lean protein, healthy fats, and a range of vitamins and minerals.

AIP Crab Cakes

AIP Crab Cakes are a tasty and healthy seafood meal suited for the Autoimmune Protocol (AIP) diet. This meal typically comprises crab flesh, a blend of spices, egg, and a binder such as mashed sweet potato or plantain. The batter is then molded into cakes and cooked or pan-fried till golden brown.

The result is a crispy surface and a supple, juicy inside with a delightful crab taste. Some varieties of AIP Crab Cakes may include the addition of herbs and spices, such as parsley, green onions, or Old Bay seasoning, for extra taste. The cakes may be served with dipping sauces or a salad for a complete meal. Overall, this meal is a tasty and nutritious alternative for individuals following the AIP diet since it includes lean protein, healthy fats, and a range of vitamins and minerals.

AIP Clam Chowder

AIP Clam Chowder is a rich and tasty soup that is suited for the Autoimmune Protocol (AIP) diet. This recipe is produced by cooking clams in a flavorful broth made from AIP-compliant ingredients such as coconut milk, onion, celery, garlic, and herbs.

The broth is then thickened with a blend of arrowroot powder or another AIP-compliant thickener, and the clams are reintroduced back to the soup to boil until they are soft. Some varieties of AIP Clam Chowder may include the addition of diced potatoes or other vegetables, such as carrots or turnips, for extra texture and taste.

The final soup is creamy and comforting, with an excellent saline taste from the clams. It is a terrific alternative for a comfortable and satisfying dinner since it includes lean protein, healthy fats, and a range of vitamins and minerals.

AIP Clam Chowder may be eaten on its own or with a side of crusty bread or crackers for a complete meal. Overall, this recipe is a beautiful and healthy alternative for people following the AIP diet searching for a savory and soothing soup option.

AIP Grilled Salmon

AIP Grilled Salmon is a tasty and healthy dinner consistent with the autoimmune diet. This recipe marries salmon filets in various AIP-friendly ingredients like olive oil, lemon juice, fresh herbs like basil or dill, and spices like sea salt and black pepper. The salmon is then cooked until it is soft and juicy, with a crispy exterior.

This meal is an excellent dose of omega-3 fatty acids, which are necessary for keeping a healthy heart, lowering inflammation, and strengthening the immune system. It is also rich in protein, vitamins B12 and D, and minerals like magnesium and potassium.

To make this recipe even tastier, add additional AIP-friendly vegetables to the grill, such as asparagus, zucchini, or bell peppers. Serve with a serving of roasted sweet potatoes or a green salad for a balanced and fulfilling supper.

AIP Lobster Bisque

AIP Lobster Bisque is a rich and flavorful soup compliant with the autoimmune diet. This dish simmers lobster shells in a broth of AIP-friendly ingredients such as coconut milk, vegetables like carrots, onions, and celery, and spices like sea salt and thyme. The mixture is then pureed until smooth, and chunks of cooked lobster meat are added back.

This dish is an excellent source of protein, healthy fats, and nutrients such as iron, magnesium, and calcium. It is also low in carbohydrates, making it an ideal option for people following a low-carb or paleo diet.

To make this dish even more satisfying, you can add some diced root vegetables, such as parsnips or turnips, to the soup while it simmers. Serve with a piece of crusty grain-free bread or a simple green salad for a comforting and delicious meal.

Recipes for vegetarian and vegan options

The Autoimmune Protocol (AIP) is a restrictive diet that eliminates certain foods that can trigger autoimmune reactions and inflammation. However, despite the restrictions, a variety of delicious and nutritious vegetarian and vegan options can be enjoyed on the AIP diet. Here are a few examples:

AIP Stuffed Bell Peppers: Bell peppers are stuffed with a combination of healthy vegetables including zucchini, eggplant, and mushrooms, along with spices and herbs for taste.

AIP Eggplant Parmesan: This recipe comprises slices of eggplant coated with coconut flour and then roasted till crispy. The eggplant is then covered with tomato sauce and served with a side of roasted veggies.

AIP Vegetable Stir-Fry: A medley of veggies, including broccoli, carrots, and onions, is stir-fried with ginger, garlic, and coconut aminos to produce a tasty savory meal.

AIP Roasted Vegetable Salad: A variety of veggies including carrots, beets, and sweet potatoes are roasted till soft and then combined with greens, herbs, and a vinaigrette dressing to make a delectable salad.

AIP Vegan "Meatballs": Lentils or chickpeas are combined with herbs and spices to produce delectable vegan "meatballs." These are then baked or sautéed and served with roasted vegetables or a salad.

By including a variety of vegetarian and vegan alternatives in their meal plans, persons following the AIP diet may enjoy a range of tastes and textures while still adhering to the principles of the AIP diet.

AIP Stuffed Bell Peppers

Stuffed bell peppers are a popular and tasty vegetarian meal that can be compatible with the Autoimmune Protocol (AIP) diet by adding a few tweaks. The cuisine often comprises bell peppers hollowed out and filled with various ingredients, such as vegetables, cereals, and meat.

For AIP compliance, you would need to avoid utilizing nightshade vegetables (such as tomatoes and peppers) and grains (such as rice or quinoa) (such as rice or quinoa). You may still have a great and healthy dinner by choosing substitute components that are AIP-friendly. For example, you may load the bell peppers with a combination of sweet potatoes, mushrooms, and herbs or with a mixture of minced beef, veggies, and spices.

Once you have prepared the filling, you stuff the hollowed-out bell peppers, place them in a baking dish, and bake in the oven until they are tender and the filling is heated. The result is flavorful and satisfying, nutrient-dense, and easy to digest. Whether you are following the AIP diet for health reasons or want to enjoy a delicious and healthy meal, stuffed bell peppers are a great option.

AIP Eggplant Parmesan

AIP Eggplant Parmesan is a tasty vegetarian recipe that fulfills the autoimmune protocol diet recommendations. It's a healthier version of the classic Italian meal prepared with eggplant slices that are breaded and fried, stacked with tomato sauce and cheese, and then baked in the oven until crispy and melted.

To make the recipe AIP-compliant, the eggplant slices are frequently baked instead of fried, and the cheese is substituted with a dairy-free replacement. The sauce is created with canned tomatoes, spices, and herbs and occasionally incorporates coconut cream or other dairy-free options. The outcome is a rich, warming dish that's excellent for a substantial supper.

AIP Vegetable Stir-Fry

AIP Vegetable Stir-Fry is a tasty and healthy recipe that anyone can enjoy following the autoimmune protocol (AIP) diet. This meal often consists of a variety of veggies stir-fried in a skillet using AIP-compliant oils, such as coconut oil or olive oil, and seasoned with AIP-friendly herbs and spices, such as garlic, ginger, and turmeric.

Some common veggies used in AIP stir-fries are carrots, bell peppers, zucchini, broccoli, and mushrooms. The veggies may be sliced and stir-fried until they are crisp-tender and then served over a bed of cauliflower rice or another grain-free substitute.

The advantages of AIP Vegetable Stir-Fry include the fact that it is a handy and fast meal, it is complete with vitamins and minerals from the different veggies, and it is adaptable to suit individual preferences and nutritional requirements. Additionally, since it is manufactured without gluten, wheat, or dairy, it is an excellent alternative for individuals with autoimmune diseases or other dietary sensitivities.

AIP Roasted Vegetable Salad

The AIP Roasted Vegetable Salad is a tasty and healthy recipe that is great for anyone following the autoimmune protocol diet. This meal is produced by roasting various veggies in the oven until they are soft and slightly browned. The roasted veggies may contain a blend of root vegetables such as carrots, sweet potatoes, and beets, as well as cruciferous vegetables like broccoli and cauliflower.

Once the veggies are roasted, they are blended with greens such as arugula or spinach and a tasty dressing created from ingredients like olive oil, lemon juice, and herbs. The roasted veggies make a deep, earthy taste and texture that compliments the soft greens and acidic dressing.

This dish is a terrific alternative for a light supper or as a side dish to complement a protein-rich main entrée. It is also a fantastic method to receive a range of nutrients, including vitamins, minerals, and fiber, in one meal. Whether you are following the autoimmune protocol diet or just searching for a nutritious and tasty dinner alternative, the AIP Roasted Vegetable Salad is sure to be a favorite!

AIP Vegan "Meatballs"

AIP Vegan "Meatballs" are a terrific choice for folks who are following the autoimmune protocol diet and are seeking a meat-free alternative. These meatballs are typically cooked using components compatible with the AIP diet, such as ground nuts, seeds, or root vegetables, and are seasoned with spices and herbs.

The texture and taste of these meatballs are typically identical to regular meatballs, but they are considerably healthier and more nutrient-dense. They may be eaten as a main meal or as a side dish and can be paired with several AIP-compliant sauces and side dishes. Some popular varieties of AIP vegan meatballs include meatballs prepared with ground almonds or sunflower seeds or from roasted carrots or sweet potatoes. These recipes are not only tasty, but they also offer the body with necessary minerals, fiber, and healthy fats.

Recipes for stews, soups, and casseroles

Stews, soups, and casseroles are warm, cozy foods that are great for more extraordinary times. These recipes may be readily changed on the AIP diet to satisfy dietary limitations while offering diverse tastes and ingredients. Some popular items in AIP-friendly stews, soups, and casseroles are root vegetables, leafy greens, and meat or seafood. Here are some examples of AIP-compliant dishes in this category:

AIP Beef Stew: This substantial recipe is composed of delicate pieces of beef, carrots, onions, and garlic, all cooked in a tasty broth.

AIP Chicken Soup: This traditional soup is created with chicken, onions, carrots, celery, and spices. It's a soothing and hearty dinner that's excellent for when you're feeling under the weather.

AIP Sweet Potato Casserole: This casserole is created with sweet potatoes, coconut milk, and spices, and it's a tasty and healthful alternative to typical sweet potato recipes.

AIP Seafood Chowder: This creamy and tasty chowder is created with salmon, shrimp, and clams, and it's a fantastic way to get in your daily amount of seafood.

AIP Vegetable Soup: This soup is prepared with various veggies, including carrots, celery, and leafy greens, and it's a fantastic way to get in your daily allotment of vegetables.

When creating stews, soups, and casseroles on the AIP diet, it's vital to use items consistent with the dietary limitations and avoid using substances like grains, dairy, and processed foods. With ingenuity, it's easy to produce tasty and gratifying recipes that follow the AIP diet.

AIP Beef Stew

AIP Beef Stew is a rich and nutritious meal that can be adapted to comply with the Autoimmune Protocol (AIP) diet. AIP Beef Stew is cooked using AIP-compatible ingredients, such as grass-fed beef, root vegetables (e.g., carrots, sweet potatoes), onions, garlic, herbs (e.g., rosemary, thyme), and a compliant stock or broth. To create an AIP Beef Stew, you start by browning the beef in a large pot or Dutch oven, then sautéing the onions and garlic. The remaining ingredients are added and cooked until the meat is done and the veggies are soft. The final product is a warm and comforting meal filled with flavor and nutrients.

AIP Chicken Soup

AIP Chicken Soup is a soothing and nutritious recipe that is excellent for individuals following the Autoimmune Protocol (AIP) diet. AIP Chicken Soup is produced with nutrient-dense ingredients that are both tasty and useful for persons with autoimmune illnesses. To create AIP Chicken Soup, you will need items such as:

- Chicken breasts or thighs
- Onion
- Carrots

- Celery
- Garlic
- Ginger
- Bone broth
- Coconut oil
- Salt and pepper

Fresh herbs such as parsley or cilantro

To create the soup, you will first sauté the onions, carrots, and celery in coconut oil until they are softened. Then, add the garlic and ginger and simmer for an additional minute. Next, add the chicken and cook until it is browned on both sides. Pour in the chicken soup and bring the soup to a boil. Turn down the heat and let it simmer for about 20 minutes or until the chicken is fully cooked. Finally, season the soup with salt and pepper and add fresh herbs.

AIP Chicken Soup is a delicious and comforting dish that can be enjoyed for lunch or dinner. It's also a wonderful alternative for meal preparation, since it can be stored in the refrigerator for up to 5 days or in the freezer for up to 3 months. Additionally, the soup can be easily customized with additional ingredients, such as sweet potatoes or turnips, to add more flavor and variety.

AIP Sweet Potato Casserole

AIP Sweet Potato Casserole is a tasty and soothing recipe consistent with the autoimmune protocol (AIP) diet. It is produced with sweet potatoes as the primary component and additional ingredients such as coconut milk, coconut flour, and spices. This recipe is excellent for a holiday feast or a comfortable weekday supper.

To create AIP Sweet Potato Casserole, you must first roast the sweet potatoes until they are cooked and then mash them. Next, mix the coconut milk and spices, then transfer the mixture to a baking dish. The final step is to bake the casserole until it is hot and bubbly.

When creating this recipe, it's vital to utilize AIP-compliant items, such as coconut flour and coconut milk, instead of wheat flour and cow's milk. Additionally, you may toss in other ingredients like raisins or almonds to make the meal even more savory and gratifying.

This AIP Sweet Potato Casserole is a tasty and healthful alternative to classic sweet potato casseroles, making it a perfect choice for anyone following the AIP diet.

AIP Seafood Chowder

AIP Seafood Chowder is a soup cooked with seafood and vegetables that are in keeping with the autoimmune protocol (AIP) diet. This soup is frequently cooked with fish, shrimp, scallops, clams, and vegetables like carrots, leeks, onions, and celery. The ingredients are cooked in a broth prepared from fish stock or a blend of coconut milk and water. To make this soup AIP-compliant, the elements should be free from nightshade vegetables, grains, dairy, nuts, and seeds. Herbs and spices that are permitted for the AIP diet, such as thyme, parsley, and bay leaves, may be added to give flavor to the soup. This dish is a healthy and substantial alternative for persons following the AIP diet and is commonly eaten as a main meal or as a beginning.

AIP Vegetable Soup

AIP Vegetable Soup is a healthy and soothing recipe that is excellent for the autoimmune protocol (AIP) diet. It is cooked with a range of healthy, AIP-compliant ingredients filled with nutrients, such as fresh veggies, bone broth, coconut milk, and spices. This meal is often low in lectins, gluten, and other inflammatory substances, making it a suitable option for individuals following the AIP diet.

To create AIP Vegetable Soup, you'll start by sautéing garlic and onions in a large soup pot. Next, you'll put in chopped veggies such as carrots, celery, sweet potatoes and spices like thyme, bay leaves, and salt. The veggies will cook for several minutes until they are somewhat softened, then you'll put in bone broth and coconut milk and bring the dish to a boil. Let the soup boil for a bit until the veggies are thoroughly cooked, and then serve hot.

This meal is adaptable, and you may alter it according to your taste preferences or the items you have on hand. For example, you may add protein-rich foods like shredded chicken or chopped sausage or use various veggies, such as squash or green beans, to provide variety. Overall, AIP Vegetable Soup is a quick, tasty, and healthy dish that is great for anybody following the autoimmune protocol.

Chapter Six

Sides and Sauces

Recipes for AIP-friendly veggies dishes

AIP-friendly vegetable meals are a crucial component of an autoimmune protocol diet since they contain critical nutrients and assist in encouraging recovery. Here are some popular AIP-compliant recipes for vegetable dishes:

Roasted Root Vegetables: This recipe comprises sweet potatoes, carrots, and parsnips, roasted to perfection with herbs like rosemary and thyme.

AIP "Fried Rice": This recipe utilizes grated veggies like cauliflower, carrots, and onion, sautéed in coconut oil, to make a "rice" like a meal AIP-compliant.

AIP Stuffed Zucchini: Zucchini boats are stuffed with ground beef, diced veggies, and seasonings, then baked until soft.

AIP-friendly Ratatouille: This famous French recipe comprises a combination of sautéed veggies, including eggplant, zucchini, bell peppers, and tomatoes, cooked together with herbs and spices.

AIP Sweet Potato & Carrot Mash: A simple and warm side dish prepared with boiling sweet potatoes and carrots, mashed together with coconut cream, olive oil, and spices.

These are just a few examples of AIP-friendly vegetable meals. The idea is to concentrate on utilizing fresh, healthy foods and to experiment with various ingredients and cooking ways to discover what works for you.

Recipes for AIP-compliant sauces and dressings

The autoimmune protocol (AIP) is a dietary strategy that avoids specific items known to increase inflammation and may provoke autoimmune symptoms. This includes processed foods, refined sugars, grains, legumes, dairy, and nightshade vegetables.

Sauces and dressings play a significant role in improving the taste and texture of meals. To ensure they are AIP-compliant, it's vital to eliminate additives like vinegar, soy sauce, and processed oils. Here are some recipes for AIP-friendly sauces and dressings:

AIP Mayo: This mayonnaise is created with coconut milk, lemon juice, and avocado oil. It's an excellent alternative to regular mayo, which typically includes vinegar or other non-AIP components.

AIP Pesto: This pesto is created with fresh basil, garlic, pine nuts, and extra virgin olive oil. It's a tasty and flexible sauce that may be used in several recipes.

AIP Ranch Dressing: This dressing is created with coconut milk, lemon juice, and herbs. It's a terrific alternative to classic ranch dressing, which typically includes dairy and other non-AIP components.

AIP BBQ Sauce: This sauce is prepared with tomatoes, honey, and spices. It's a terrific alternative for grilling or marinating meats and veggies.

AIP Tahini Dressing: This dressing is made with tahini, lemon juice, and garlic. It's a delicious addition to salads, vegetables, and grain-free wraps.

These are just a few examples of the many AIP-compliant sauces and dressings that can be made at home. Using fresh, whole ingredients and avoiding non-AIP ingredients makes it possible to create delicious and nutritious sauces and condiments that support the healing process and improve overall health.

Recipes for fermented veggies

Fermented vegetables are a cornerstone of the autoimmune protocol (AIP) diet since they offer a rich supply of probiotics and improve gut health. The fermentation process includes employing microbes to break down plant sugars and carbs, generating valuable enzymes, vitamins, and amino acids. Here are a few recipes for AIP-compliant fermented vegetables:

Classic Sauerkraut: This basic recipe utilizes cabbage and salt, allowing the natural fermentation process to proceed. Cut cabbage, knead it with salt, and store it in a jar, allowing about an inch of headroom. Cover with a cloth and let ferment for several days, then keep in the refrigerator.

Pickled Carrots: These sweet and tangy carrots are a terrific complement to any dinner. Combine shredded carrots with salt, let lie for a few hours, then put into a jar with spices such as cumin, coriander, and mustard seeds. Fill with a brine prepared from water, salt, and vinegar, then let ferment for several days.

Fermented Beets: These spicy, somewhat sour beets complement salads or as a side dish. Cut and blend with cinnamon, ginger, and allspice, then let ferment for several days in a brine prepared from water, salt, and vinegar.

Kimchi: This traditional Korean meal is created from a blend of cabbage, radish, ginger, and spices and is a mainstay of the AIP diet. Cut the items, combine them with a spicy spice mixture, and let ferment for several days.

Remember, while creating fermented veggies, utilizing high-quality products and observing strict food safety standards is crucial. If you discover any symptoms of spoiling, such as mold or odd scents, trash the batch and start again.

Recipes for pickles and chutneys

Pickles and chutneys are popular condiments in many cultures and may be produced in several ways using various vegetables and spices. Pickling is a way of preserving food by keeping it in an acidic solution, commonly vinegar. In contrast, chutneys are usually created with a mixture of spices, herbs, and fruit cooked until thickened.

Here are some AIP-compliant recipes for pickles and chutneys:

AIP Pickles:

Cut cucumbers into thin slices and set them in a dish.

In a separate basin, mix up equal parts apple cider vinegar and water, and add salt and a few spices like dill, garlic, or black peppercorns.

Ladle the vinegar slurry over the cucumbers and let them rest for at least 30 minutes before eating.

AIP Chutney:

In a food processor, blend fresh herbs like mint and cilantro, fresh or dried fruit like dates or raisins, spices like ginger and turmeric, and a little water.

Blend everything until it makes a smooth sauce. Serve the chutney as a condiment with meats or vegetables, or use it as a dipping sauce.
Remember, while creating pickles or chutneys, observing food safety requirements is crucial to minimize deterioration and the danger of foodborne disease.

Chapter Seven

Sweets and Treats

AIP-compliant sweeteners and ingredients

When following the autoimmune protocol (AIP), it's crucial to pick both healthful and supportive components of gut health. Many typical sweets and additives might be inflammatory, so choosing AIP-compliant alternatives is vital. Some of the most prevalent AIP-compliant sweeteners include:

Honey is a natural sweetener rich in antioxidants, enzymes, and minerals and well-tolerated by many persons following AIP.

Maple syrup: made from the sap of sugar maples, this sweetener is packed in antioxidants, minerals, and vitamins and is an AIP-friendly alternative to processed sweets.

Coconut sugar: a low-glycemic sweetener derived from the sap of coconut palms, coconut sugar is rich in vitamins, minerals, and antioxidants, making it a fantastic option for AIP.

Date paste: produced from dates, this natural sweetener is abundant in fiber, vitamins, and minerals and is a flexible alternative to processed sugars.

Other products regularly utilized in AIP cuisine include coconut oil, olive oil, coconut flour, cassava flour, and arrowroot starch. These substances replace wheat flour, cornstarch, and other grains since they are free from gluten and other grains that might cause inflammation in persons with autoimmune illnesses.

Additionally, coconut oil and olive oil are fantastic sources of healthy fats that help promote gut health and general well-being.

Maple syrup

Maple syrup is a sweetener manufactured from the sap of maple trees. It is widely used as a natural alternative to refined sugar. The liquid is gathered from the trees in the spring and then boiled down to concentrate the natural sugars. The result is a thick, amber-colored syrup that has a unique, sweet, and somewhat earthy taste.

Maple syrup is an essential component in many classic American and Canadian cuisine and is widely used as a topping for pancakes and waffles. It may also be used in baking recipes such as cakes, muffins, biscuits, sauces, and marinades for meat and fish meals.

There are numerous grades of maple syrup, which vary in color and taste. The darker the syrup, the greater the flavor. Grade A syrups are lighter in color and have a gentler, sweeter taste, while Grade B syrups are darker and have a stronger, more robust flavor.

It's crucial to remember that although maple syrup is regarded as a better option than refined sugar, it still includes a significant quantity of natural sugars and should be used in moderation as part of a balanced diet.

Coconut sugar

Coconut sugar, commonly known as coconut palm sugar, is a sweetener made from the sap of the coconut palm tree. It is created by boiling the juice of the tree until it hardens and crystallizes, generating a granular product similar in look and texture to brown sugar. Coconut sugar is considered a healthier option than other sweeteners, such as white sugar, owing to its lower glycemic index and increased vitamin content. It includes vitamins and minerals, including potassium, magnesium, zinc, iron, and B vitamins.

Coconut sugar may be used as a one-to-one substitute for white sugar in many recipes. Its flavor is typically akin to brown sugar with a somewhat nutty, caramel-like taste. Because it is lightly processed, coconut sugar keeps some of the natural aromas and nutrients of the coconut palm sap, which sets it apart from other refined sweeteners. It is compatible with the Autoimmune Protocol (AIP) and may be used in AIP-friendly recipes as a sweetener.

Date paste

Date paste is a sweet, thick, and spreadable substance produced from dates. It is a natural sweetener in several AIP-compliant dishes, including baked products, smoothies, and sauces. To make date paste, dates are first soaked in water to soften them, then pureed into a smooth purée. Some recipes may ask for additional ingredients such as water, vanilla extract, or lemon juice to aid the blending process. Date paste tastes caramel and is a beautiful alternative to refined sugar in AIP-compliant dishes. It also serves as a good source of fiber and essential vitamins and minerals. However, it is crucial to remember that date paste, like other sweeteners, should be used in moderation as part of a balanced diet.

Recipes for sweets

Here are some recipes for AIP-friendly desserts:

AIP Banana Bread: Made with almond flour and coconut flour and sweetened with dates, this banana bread is a tasty and healthier alternative to typical baked products.

AIP Berry Crumble: This meal is created with a combination of frozen berries, coconut flour, coconut sugar, and coconut oil, and topped with a crumble made from almond flour and coconut oil.

AIP Ice Cream: This dairy-free ice cream is created with coconut cream, coconut sugar, and your choice of flavorings, such as vanilla extract or chocolate powder.

AIP Lemon Treats: These lemon bars are prepared with almond flour and coconut flour and sweetened with maple syrup. They are acidic and delicious, with a crumbly crust and a creamy lemon filling.

AIP Apple Crisp: This recipe is created with thinly sliced apples, cinnamon, nutmeg, and a topping made from almond flour, coconut sugar, and coconut oil.

These are just a handful of the numerous AIP-friendly dessert alternatives available. When preparing sweets on the AIP diet, it's vital to utilize permitted sweeteners and ingredients

and avoid processed meals, dairy, gluten, and other inflammatory substances.
Recipes for baked foods

Baked goods are a mainstay in many people's diets. On the autoimmune protocol (AIP), there are many possibilities for preparing tasty baked goodies that are consistent with the elimination phase of the diet. Some common AIP-compliant ingredients used in baking include coconut flour, almond flour, tapioca flour, and arrowroot flour.

These flours may be used to produce cakes, cookies, bread, and other baked products. Additionally, AIP-friendly sweeteners like maple syrup, honey, and coconut sugar may be used instead of regular sugar. Eggs are also a regularly utilized component in AIP baked products since they give structure and help bind things together.

Examples of AIP-compliant baked items include:

- Coconut Flour Banana Bread
- Almond Flour Blueberry Muffins
- Tapioca Flour Pie Crust
- Arrowroot Flour Waffles
- Coconut Flour Carrot Cake
- Almond Flour Lemon Bars

When baking AIP-compliant baked products, it's vital to pay attention to the ingredients and ensure they are compatible with the autoimmune protocol. Additionally, some individuals on the AIP may need to experiment with various flours and sweeteners to determine what works best for them and their unique autoimmune issues.

Recipes for sweets and snacks

Recipes for desserts and snacks on the autoimmune protocol (AIP) often employ items consistent with the protocol's dietary limitations. Some standard components in AIP desserts and snacks include coconut flour, cassava flour, coconut oil, coconut cream, and different sweeteners such as maple syrup, honey, and dates. Some examples of AIP-friendly desserts and snacks include:

AIP Banana Bread: Made with coconut flour, almond flour, bananas, eggs, and other AIP-compliant ingredients, this bread delivers a delicious and comforting snack.

AIP "Oatmeal" Cookies: These cookies are created with a blend of nuts and seeds mixed into the flour and sweetened with a compliant sweetener.

AIP Fruit Leather: A combination of pureed fruit, spices, and a compliant sweetener, spread thin and dried to produce a chewy fruit snack.

AIP Trail Mix: A blend of nuts, seeds, dried fruit, and occasionally chocolate chips, this is a terrific snack to take on the move.

AIP Energy Bites: These are little, ball-shaped snacks prepared with nuts, seeds, dried fruit, and spices, frequently kept together with nut butter or coconut oil.

It's crucial to remember that although these sweets and snacks may be created using AIP-compliant foods, they should still be taken in moderation since they are still rich in calories and may contribute to weight gain.

Chapter Eight

Conclusion and Resources

Tips for success on the AIP diet

The AIP diet may be a challenging yet beneficial nutritional strategy. To optimize your chances of success, consider the following tips:

Plan your meals: This will help ensure that you always have AIP-compliant products on hand and may simplify meal prep.

Shop smart: Stock up on AIP-friendly products like fresh vegetables, fruits, and meats, and avoid processed and packaged meals.

Get creative in the kitchen: Experiment with new AIP-friendly dishes to keep things exciting and minimize monotony.

Cook at home: Preparing your own meals is the most excellent method to guarantee that you follow the AIP diet completely and avoid hidden additives that may provoke autoimmune symptoms.

Listen to your body: Pay attention to how various meals impact you and make modifications as required.

Be bold and ask for help: If you're feeling overwhelmed or need assistance, reach out to others who are following the AIP diet or to a healthcare professional versed in the AIP diet.

Be patient and persistent: The AIP diet may require a considerable lifestyle shift and might take time to see effects. Stick with it, and you will likely experience general health and well-being benefits.

Remember, everyone's body is different, and what works for one person may not work for another. It's vital to work closely with your healthcare provider to identify what's best for you and to ensure you are adequately supported along the journey.

How to integrate AIP into your lifestyle

Incorporating the AIP diet into your lifestyle involves some planning and preparation but can be a gratifying and enjoyable experience. Here are some recommendations to assist you in making the transition:

Start with simple changes: Begin by making tiny, progressive modifications to your diet rather than attempting to overhaul everything completely.

Plan ahead: Meal planning and preparation are essential to success on the AIP diet. Make a plan for the week, and fill your pantry and refrigerator with AIP-friendly items.

Get creative in the kitchen: Try new dishes and experiment with AIP-compliant items to discover your preferred meals.

Read labels carefully: Read the labels of packaged items carefully to verify they match AIP requirements. Avoid processed meals and search for lightly processed ones.

Find AIP-friendly eateries: Research places that provide AIP-compliant alternatives, or try cooking at home more regularly.

Connect with other AIP enthusiasts: Seek out support from people following the AIP diet. Join online forums, attend local events, or find a companion to exchange recipes and experiences with.

Stay patient: Change takes time, so trust the process. If you mess up or battle with cravings, try to be gentle to yourself and get back on track as quickly as possible.

By following these suggestions, you may effectively adopt the AIP diet into your lifestyle and enjoy its advantages.

Resources for additional information and assistance

Several resources are available for people searching for more excellent information and assistance on the AIP (Autoimmune Protocol) diet. Some of the more frequent and valuable resources include:

Books: Various books on the market explain the AIP diet in-depth, including "The Autoimmune Protocol Handbook" by Mickey Trescott and "The Healing Kitchen" by Alaena Haber and Sarah Ballantyne.

Websites: Various websites give information and resources for the AIP diet, including autoimmune-protocol.com, paleo autoimmune protocol.com, and phoenixhelix.com.

Social Media: There are several Facebook groups, Twitter accounts, and Instagram profiles devoted to the AIP community, which may be a terrific resource for support, advice, and recipes.

Practitioners: It might be good to work with a practitioner with expertise in the AIP diet, such as a nutritionist, dietitian, or functional medicine specialist. They can help you adjust the diet to your unique requirements and give direction and assistance.

Online Groups: There are online communities and forums, such as Reddit and the AIP Community on Facebook, where users may ask questions and interact with others following the AIP diet.

It is crucial to note that everyone's experience with the AIP diet is unique, and it may take time to determine what works best for you. However, with the aid of these materials, you may boost your chances of success and make the transition to the AIP diet a pleasant one.

Conclusion and last remarks.

In conclusion, the Autoimmune Protocol (AIP) is a stringent elimination diet that may help patients manage autoimmune disorders and enhance their overall health and well-being. The AIP diet removes numerous major allergens and inflammatory foods, including grains, legumes, dairy, sugar, and processed foods. Instead, it emphasizes nutrient-dense, whole foods such as vegetables, fruits, meats, and healthy fats.

The AIP diet may be tough to follow, but careful planning and preparation can be a very effective strategy to decrease inflammation and relieve symptoms. It's vital to remember that the AIP diet is not a one-size-fits-all strategy, and it's necessary to engage with a healthcare expert to find the optimal plan for your unique requirements.

Numerous resources are available for anyone interested in following the AIP diet, including cookbooks, online groups, and websites that give information, support, and recipes. It's also good to connect with people who are following the AIP diet, since they may provide direction and support during the process.

Regarding concluding comments, the AIP diet is a vital tool for controlling autoimmune disorders, but it's crucial to approach it with care and seek expert supervision. It's also essential to be patient and persistent since it may take many weeks or months to realize the full advantages of the AIP diet. Remember to concentrate on fueling your body with nutrient-dense, whole meals and to be gentle and patient with yourself during the process.